Navigating Morning Sickness in Pregnancy:

Causes, Treatments, and Empowerment

Katharine W.

Table of contents

1. Introduction
2. Understanding Morning Sickness
3. Unveiling Hormonal Triggers
4. Genetic Correlations
5. Clinical Insights and Research
6. Future Prospects and Considerations
7. Empowering Expectant Parents
8. Conclusion

Introduction:

The Phenomenon of Morning Sickness:

Understanding Nausea and Vomiting in Pregnancy

Morning sickness, a common yet complex experience during pregnancy, manifests as nausea and occasional vomiting, impacting a significant percentage of expectant individuals. This phenomenon, occurring predominantly during the first trimester but sometimes persisting throughout pregnancy, varies widely in intensity and duration among different individuals.

Understanding the Experience:

The onset of morning sickness can be unsettling and challenging for many expectant parents. Despite its misleading name, this discomfort can strike at any time of the day, disrupting daily routines and causing distress. The prevalence of morning sickness, affecting around 80% of pregnant individuals, signifies the importance of delving deeper into its causes and impacts.

Factors at Play:

While the exact cause of morning sickness remains elusive, hormonal fluctuations, especially increased levels of human chorionic gonadotropin (hCG) and estrogen during early pregnancy, are widely believed to contribute to this condition. Additionally, the role of psychological, genetic, and dietary factors in exacerbating or alleviating morning sickness adds layers of complexity to its understanding.

Impact on Expectant Parents:

Beyond its physical symptoms, morning sickness can have profound emotional and social implications. Coping with persistent nausea, disrupted eating patterns, and the challenge of maintaining daily activities can take a toll on an individual's well-being and mental health during this crucial phase.

Navigating the Journey:

Understanding the pervasive nature of morning sickness is crucial for expectant parents and healthcare providers alike. Unraveling the intricacies of this phenomenon opens pathways for effective coping strategies, treatment options, and empowering expectant individuals to navigate this challenging yet common aspect of pregnancy.

Impact on Expectant Parents: Understanding the physical, emotional, and social implications of morning sickness

Physical Effects:

- Dehydration and Nutritional Concerns: Severe morning sickness, especially when accompanied by frequent vomiting, can lead to dehydration and nutritional deficiencies. This can affect the health of the parent and potentially impact the developing fetus.

- Fatigue and Discomfort: Constant nausea and vomiting can lead to fatigue and general discomfort, making it challenging to carry out daily activities or work efficiently.

Emotional Toll:

- Stress and Anxiety: Dealing with persistent nausea and vomiting can cause stress and anxiety, affecting the emotional well-being of expectant parents. This emotional strain may exacerbate feelings of uncertainty and fear about the pregnancy.
- Mood Swings: Hormonal changes coupled with the physical discomfort of morning sickness can contribute to mood swings and emotional instability.

Social Implications:

- Impact on Daily Life: Severe morning sickness may interfere with one's ability to work, attend social gatherings, or fulfill responsibilities, leading to isolation and feelings of being disconnected from normal routines.
- Support Networks: Having a strong support system comprising family, friends, or support groups can significantly mitigate the challenges posed by morning sickness. However, lack of understanding or support from others might exacerbate the emotional toll.

Coping Strategies:

- Seeking Medical Advice: Consulting healthcare professionals for guidance and support can alleviate concerns and provide personalized strategies to manage morning sickness effectively.
- Open Communication: Sharing experiences and feelings with a partner, family, or friends can provide emotional relief and create a supportive environment.
- Self-care and Rest: Prioritizing self-care, including adequate rest, maintaining proper hydration, and eating small, nutritious meals, can help manage the physical and emotional impact of morning sickness.

Long-term Outlook:

- For most parents-to-be, morning sickness tends to subside as pregnancy progresses, usually by the second trimester. However, for a small percentage, symptoms might persist throughout pregnancy.

Understanding the multifaceted impact of morning sickness on expectant parents can foster empathy and support within communities, providing a more comprehensive approach to assisting those experiencing this challenging aspect of pregnancy.

Chapter 2:

Understanding Morning Sickness

Defining the Spectrum: Differentiating between typical morning sickness and severe hyperemesis gravidarum

Morning Sickness:

- Typical Occurrence: Common during the first trimester of pregnancy, affecting about 70-80% of pregnant individuals.
- Symptoms: Mild to moderate nausea, occasional vomiting, sensitivity to smells, and aversions to certain foods.
- Timing: Often occurs in the morning but can happen at any time of the day.
- Duration: Usually resolves by the second trimester.
- Management: Dietary changes, small, frequent meals, rest, over-the-counter remedies (e.g., ginger), and lifestyle adjustments are often effective.

Hyperemesis Gravidarum:

- Rare Occurrence: A severe form of morning sickness, affecting around 1-3% of pregnancies.
- Symptoms: Severe, persistent nausea, excessive vomiting multiple times a day, leading to dehydration and weight loss.

- Timing: Continues throughout pregnancy and may worsen as it progresses.
- Impact: Impairs daily functioning, leads to emotional distress, severe fatigue, and may require hospitalization.
- Treatment: Requires medical intervention, including hospitalization for intravenous fluids, anti-nausea medications, and close monitoring by healthcare professionals.
- Long-term Management: May persist throughout pregnancy, needing ongoing medical care and support.

<u>Potential Risks:</u>

- For the Parent: Dehydration, nutritional deficiencies, and emotional strain.
- For the Baby: Possible complications due to severe dehydration and malnutrition, impacting fetal growth and development.

Understanding the differences between morning sickness and hyperemesis gravidarum is essential for prompt identification, appropriate medical care, and support for expectant parents experiencing severe symptoms during pregnancy.

Global Prevalence: Examining the prevalence rates and variations of morning sickness worldwide

- Varied Incidence Rates: Morning sickness, a common occurrence during pregnancy, varies in its prevalence across different populations and geographic regions.
- Incidence Rates: Studies suggest that approximately 70-80% of pregnant individuals experience some form of morning sickness.
- Geographic Variations: Prevalence rates of morning sickness can differ significantly based on geographical locations, cultural practices, and socioeconomic factors.
- Cultural Influence: Cultural differences may influence the reporting and management of morning sickness. Some cultures might have specific remedies or traditional practices to alleviate symptoms.

Regional and Demographic Factors:

- Higher Prevalence in Certain Regions: Studies indicate higher rates of morning sickness in Western countries compared to some non-Western regions.

- Demographic Variances: Factors such as age, socioeconomic status, dietary habits, and access to healthcare can impact the incidence and severity of morning sickness within populations.

<u>Research and Reporting:</u>

- Global Studies: Research on morning sickness prevalence spans various countries, aiming to understand its frequency and impact on expectant parents worldwide.
- Reporting Discrepancies: Discrepancies in reporting might exist due to varying definitions of morning sickness and differences in survey methodologies across studies.
- Data Collection Challenges: Access to healthcare, cultural perceptions, and varying pregnancy experiences can make it challenging to gather consistent data on morning sickness prevalence globally.

<u>Impact on Public Health:</u>

- Awareness and Support: Understanding the global prevalence of morning sickness is crucial for healthcare systems to provide adequate support and resources for pregnant individuals.

- Improving Care: Knowledge of prevalence rates across diverse populations can aid in developing targeted interventions and support systems for managing morning sickness.

Chapter 3:

Unveiling Hormonal Triggers

Fetal Hormones and Nausea: Investigating how hormones produced by the fetus contribute to the onset of morning sickness

Human Chorionic Gonadotropin (hCG):

- hCG is a hormone produced by the placenta shortly after implantation, peaking around weeks 9-10 of pregnancy before declining.
- The rapid increase in hCG levels is often associated with the onset of nausea and vomiting, particularly during the first trimester.

Theories Exploring the Role of hCG:

- Sensitivity of Maternal Body: Some studies suggest that high levels of hCG might affect the sensitivity of the maternal body to other stimuli, potentially triggering nausea and vomiting.
- Hormonal Influence: hCG might have an impact on the hypothalamus, triggering the release of hormones like estrogen and progesterone, which, in turn, could contribute to gastrointestinal changes leading to nausea.
- Evolutionary Perspective: There are theories suggesting that morning sickness might serve as a protective mechanism for the developing

fetus. By avoiding certain foods or odors that trigger nausea, the pregnant individual may protect the fetus from potentially harmful substances.

Variances and Limitations:

- While a correlation exists between hCG levels and the onset of morning sickness in some individuals, it doesn't imply direct causation. Many pregnant individuals with high hCG levels don't experience severe morning sickness, highlighting the complexity of the relationship.
- There's a lack of consistent evidence directly establishing how hCG specifically triggers nausea and vomiting. Other factors, such as genetic predisposition, lifestyle, and environmental influences, likely play significant roles

Research Challenges and Future Directions:

- Research into the relationship between fetal hormones, particularly hCG, and morning sickness is ongoing. Challenges include the complexity of hormonal interactions and the individual variability in symptom experiences.

Placental Hormones:

- The placenta, not the fetus itself, produces hormones like human chorionic gonadotropin (hCG), estrogen, and progesterone during pregnancy.

- hCG: Often associated with pregnancy, this hormone rises significantly in the early stages and is believed to play a role in nausea, possibly affecting the sensitivity of the maternal body to other stimuli.

Theoretical Connection:

- Some theories suggest that elevated levels of hCG may influence the occurrence of morning sickness. However, the exact mechanisms through which these hormones trigger nausea remain unclear.
- While hCG levels correlate with the onset of morning sickness in some cases, direct causation is yet to be established.

Alternative Perspectives:

- Other factors like genetic predisposition, sensitivity to hormonal changes, and alterations in the gastrointestinal tract due to pregnancy hormones may contribute to the development of morning sickness.
- The exact interplay between fetal hormones and maternal symptoms remains an area of ongoing research and is not solely attributed to fetal hormones' actions.

Varied Experiences:

- It's important to note that not all pregnant individuals experience morning sickness, and the severity and onset of symptoms vary widely among those who do.
- Individual differences in hormone levels and their sensitivity to hormonal changes contribute to the diverse experiences with morning sickness during pregnancy.

While fetal hormones, especially hCG, are considered a potential factor in the onset of morning sickness, further research is needed to definitively establish their specific role in causing nausea and vomiting during pregnancy.

GDF15 Significance: Analyzing the role of GDF15 hormone in triggering and managing morning sickness symptoms

What is GDF15?

- Growth Differentiation Factor 15 (GDF15) is a protein naturally produced in the body, recognized for its involvement in various physiological processes such as cell regulation, metabolism, and appetite control.
- GDF15 is secreted by various tissues and cells, including placental tissues during pregnancy.

GDF15 and Pregnancy:

- During pregnancy, levels of GDF15 in the bloodstream significantly increase, particularly in the first trimester.
- The elevation of GDF15 during pregnancy coincides with the onset of morning sickness symptoms in some individuals.

Role of GDF15 in Triggering Nausea:

- Studies suggest that heightened levels of GDF15 might influence specific brain areas responsible for inducing nausea and vomiting.
- GDF15 might affect neural pathways associated with nausea sensitivity, potentially contributing to the development of morning sickness symptoms

Exploring GDF15 for Managing Morning Sickness:

- While GDF15 is associated with the onset of morning sickness symptoms, its direct role in managing or alleviating these symptoms remains under investigation.
- Research into GDF15's actions could pave the way for potential therapies targeting its effects on the brain's nausea centers, offering novel approaches to managing severe morning sickness.

Clinical Implications and Future Studies:

- Scientists are exploring GDF15 as a potential biomarker to identify individuals at risk of severe morning sickness, such as hyperemesis gravidarum.
- Investigating GDF15's mechanisms of action could lead to the development of targeted treatments aiming to mitigate the severity of nausea and vomiting during pregnancy.

Research Limitations and Future Directions:

- While GDF15 shows promise in its association with morning sickness, further research is crucial to fully comprehend its exact role and potential therapeutic applications.
- Challenges include determining causality, understanding variations in GDF15 levels among different individuals, and exploring potential interventions based on these findings.

Chapter4:

Genetic Correlations

Genetic Associations: Exploring genetic data linking GDF15 levels pre-pregnancy to the severity of morning sickness

Pre-Pregnancy GDF15 Levels:

- Recent studies have explored the possibility of genetic links between baseline (pre-pregnancy) GDF15 levels and the severity of morning sickness experienced during pregnancy.
- Researchers have investigated whether variations in GDF15-related genes before pregnancy might predispose individuals to experiencing more severe morning sickness symptoms.

Genetic Variants and Susceptibility:
- Some genetic variants associated with higher baseline GDF15 levels have been identified in certain individuals.
- These genetic variations could potentially influence the levels of GDF15 during early pregnancy, contributing to a higher likelihood of experiencing severe morning sickness symptoms.

Research Findings:

- Preliminary research indicates that certain genetic variations linked to increased GDF15 levels prior to pregnancy might correlate with a higher risk of experiencing more severe morning sickness symptoms during gestation.
- However, these genetic associations are still being studied and need further validation across diverse populations to establish their reliability and significance.

Clinical Implications and Future Studies:

- Understanding the genetic factors influencing baseline GDF15 levels and their impact on morning sickness severity could offer valuable insights into predicting and managing severe symptoms during pregnancy.
- Further investigations are required to confirm and expand upon these genetic associations, considering factors such as ethnic diversity and the interplay of multiple genetic factors affecting GDF15 regulation.

Challenges and Continued Research:

- Challenges in genetic studies of this nature include the need for large-scale studies encompassing diverse populations, addressing potential confounding factors, and confirming the causative role of identified genetic variants.
- Longitudinal studies tracking GDF15 levels and symptom severity across pre-pregnancy and

throughout pregnancy would provide more comprehensive insights.

Individual Susceptibility: Understanding how genetic predispositions influence an individual's sensitivity to morning sickness

Variability in Susceptibility:

- Genetic factors contribute to the wide variability in how individuals experience and respond to morning sickness during pregnancy.
- Certain genetic variations influence how the body processes hormones, responds to changes in hormone levels, and regulates physiological responses, potentially impacting one's susceptibility to nausea and vomiting.

Genetic Influence on Hormonal Response:

- Genetic variations in genes responsible for hormone regulation, particularly those involved in estrogen, progesterone, and hCG metabolism, can influence an individual's sensitivity to hormonal changes during pregnancy.

- These variations may affect how the body tolerates or reacts to fluctuations in hormone levels, which can contribute to the severity and onset of morning sickness symptoms.

Gene-Environment Interactions:

- While genetic predispositions play a crucial role, environmental factors also contribute to the manifestation of morning sickness.
- Lifestyle, dietary habits, stress levels, and other environmental influences can interact with genetic factors, either exacerbating or mitigating the severity of symptoms.

Research Insights:

- Studies have identified specific genetic markers associated with an increased risk or decreased susceptibility to morning sickness.
- These genetic markers often relate to pathways involved in hormone metabolism, neurotransmitter regulation, and the body's response to stress.

Impact on Clinical Practice:

- Understanding an individual's genetic predispositions could aid healthcare providers in predicting the likelihood or severity of morning sickness.

- Tailoring care plans and offering personalized interventions based on an individual's genetic profile might help manage symptoms more effectively.

<u>Challenges and Future Research:</u>

- Unraveling the complex interplay between genetic factors, hormonal changes, and environmental influences requires extensive research.
- Longitudinal studies involving diverse populations and considering multifaceted interactions between genes and environmental factors are crucial for a comprehensive understanding.

Chapter5:

Clinical Insights and Research

Animal Studies and Clinical Trials: Discussing findings from studies testing GDF15 impact on animal models and potential implications for human treatments

Animal Model Studies:

- Animal studies, particularly in rodents, have investigated the effects of GDF15 on appetite regulation, metabolism, and nausea response.
- Research in animal models has shown that increased levels of GDF15 correlate with reduced food intake, weight loss, and changes in behavior related to nausea and vomiting.

Potential Implications for Humans:

- Animal studies suggest that manipulating GDF15 levels or its signaling pathways might influence nausea sensitivity and appetite regulation.
- These findings hint at the potential for GDF15-related interventions to modulate symptoms associated with nausea and vomiting, including those experienced during pregnancy.

Clinical Trials and Human Relevance:

- Clinical trials exploring GDF15 as a therapeutic target for conditions related to appetite control and metabolic disorders are ongoing.
- While these trials may not specifically focus on morning sickness, their findings could offer insights into the broader implications of GDF15 modulation for managing symptoms like nausea in various contexts.

Challenges and Translation to Human Treatments:

- Translating findings from animal studies to human treatments poses challenges due to differences in physiology, metabolism, and the complexity of human responses.
- The relevance of GDF15 modulation in addressing morning sickness in humans requires further research and specific clinical trials targeting this aspect of pregnancy.

Future Directions and Therapeutic Potential:

- Exploring GDF15 as a potential therapeutic target for managing nausea and vomiting during pregnancy remains an area of interest and could lead to the development of novel treatments.
- Human trials specifically designed to investigate the impact of GDF15 modulation on symptoms associated with morning sickness could provide valuable insights.

<u>Potential Therapeutic Paths: Highlighting avenues for modifying GDF15 sensitivity to mitigate morning sickness severity</u>

1. <u>GDF15 Modulation:</u>

- Pharmacological Interventions: Developing medications or therapies targeting GDF15 receptors or its signaling pathways might offer a means to modulate its effects on nausea sensitivity.
- GDF15 Inhibitors or Agonists: Investigating compounds that can either block or enhance GDF15's activity might provide avenues for managing symptoms associated with morning sickness.

2. <u>Hormone Regulation:</u>

- Hormone Balancing: Understanding the interplay between GDF15 and other pregnancy-related hormones (e.g., hCG, estrogen) could lead to approaches that balance hormonal fluctuations, potentially mitigating nausea severity.
- Targeted Hormone Therapies: Developing hormone-based therapies or interventions that

specifically address imbalances contributing to heightened GDF15 levels might offer relief from severe morning sickness.

3. <u>Nutritional Interventions:</u>

- Dietary Modifications: Exploring nutritional approaches that influence GDF15 levels or its impact on nausea sensitivity might provide non-pharmacological options for managing morning sickness.
- Supplements or Nutraceuticals: Investigating the effects of specific nutrients or supplements on GDF15 metabolism could offer potential interventions to alleviate symptoms.

4. <u>Lifestyle and Behavioral Interventions:</u>

- Stress Management: Research into stress reduction techniques or behavioral interventions that influence stress-related pathways might indirectly impact GDF15 sensitivity and alleviate morning sickness symptoms.
- Dietary and Lifestyle Changes: Promoting healthier lifestyle choices or specific dietary modifications based on GDF15-related research might aid in managing nausea severity.

5. <u>Personalized Medicine Approaches:</u>

- Genetic Profiling: Identifying genetic markers associated with heightened GDF15 sensitivity might pave the way for personalized interventions tailored to individual genetic profiles.
- Targeted Therapies: Developing treatments based on an individual's genetic predispositions, hormone levels, and other physiological markers could offer more precise and effective management of morning sickness.

<u>Challenges and Considerations:</u>

- The complexity of GDF15's actions and interactions with other physiological pathways poses challenges in developing targeted therapies.
- Ensuring safety, efficacy, and specific targeting without adverse effects on pregnancy or fetal development is crucial in the development of any therapeutic interventions.

Chapter6:

Future Prospects and Considerations

Treatment Challenges: Addressing potential risks and ethical considerations related to altering GDF15 activity

1. ### Potential Risks:

- Fetal Development: Any intervention aimed at altering GDF15 activity must consider potential effects on fetal development and growth, ensuring the safety of the unborn child.
- Unintended Side Effects: Modulating GDF15 levels or activity might lead to unintended physiological changes, affecting other bodily functions beyond nausea and vomiting.

2. ### Ethical Considerations:

- Pregnancy Safety: Interventions targeting GDF15 must prioritize the safety of both the pregnant individual and the developing fetus, raising ethical concerns regarding the risks and benefits of such interventions during gestation.
- Informed Consent: Ensuring individuals have comprehensive information about potential treatments, their risks, and uncertain outcomes is crucial for obtaining informed consent,

particularly in the context of pregnancy-related therapies.

3. <u>Complexity of GDF15:</u>

- Interconnected Pathways: GDF15 is involved in various physiological processes beyond nausea regulation. Modifying its activity might inadvertently affect other systems, necessitating a comprehensive understanding of its multifaceted roles.
- Potential Long-term Effects: Considering the long-term consequences of altering GDF15 activity is essential, especially when the interventions occur during pregnancy, which could impact not only the current gestation but also future pregnancies and the individual's health.

4. <u>Regulatory and Clinical Challenges:</u>

- Clinical Trials: Conducting clinical trials to assess the efficacy and safety of GDF15-related interventions during pregnancy raises challenges in ensuring rigorous study designs, ethical oversight, and long-term follow-up of participants.
- Regulatory Approval: Gaining regulatory approval for pregnancy-related therapies involving GDF15 modulation requires extensive

preclinical data, safety assessments, and ethical considerations, which might pose challenges in the approval process.

Altering GDF15 activity to manage morning sickness presents potential therapeutic benefits but also poses significant challenges in ensuring safety, understanding long-term effects, and navigating ethical considerations. Balancing the risks and benefits while addressing these challenges is crucial in the development of any GDF15-related treatments for pregnant individuals experiencing severe morning sickness.

Clinical Applications: Speculating on the future of treatments and research directions in managing severe morning sickness

1. Targeted Therapies:

- GDF15-Targeted Interventions: Further research might lead to the development of therapies specifically targeting GDF15 or its

signaling pathways to mitigate nausea and vomiting during pregnancy.
- Personalized Medicine Approaches: Advancements in genetic profiling could enable tailored interventions based on an individual's genetic predispositions related to GDF15 sensitivity.

2. <u>Hormone Modulation:</u>

- Hormonal Balance Interventions: Understanding hormonal interactions, especially those involving hCG, estrogen, and progesterone, could offer avenues for balancing hormone levels and managing severe morning sickness.
- Novel Hormonal Therapies: Research might unveil hormone-based therapies tailored to address imbalances contributing to heightened GDF15 levels and associated symptoms.

3. <u>Nutritional and Lifestyle Interventions:</u>

- Dietary Modifications: Further exploration of nutritional strategies influencing GDF15 levels or its effects on nausea might provide non-pharmacological options for symptom management.
- Behavioral Modifications: Advancing knowledge of stress-related pathways and their interactions with GDF15 might lead to behavioral interventions aiding in symptom alleviation.

4.Clinical Trial Advancements:

- Specific Pregnancy-Related Trials: Designing and conducting clinical trials focused explicitly on GDF15 modulation and its impact on morning sickness symptoms during pregnancy.
- Longitudinal Studies: Long-term observational studies tracking GDF15 levels and symptom severity across pre-pregnancy, throughout pregnancy, and postpartum could offer comprehensive insights.

5. Comprehensive Support Systems:

- Multidisciplinary Care: Establishing comprehensive care models involving healthcare professionals specializing in obstetrics, genetics, nutrition, and mental health to offer holistic support for individuals experiencing severe morning sickness.
- Patient Education and Support Networks: Enhancing awareness and support networks for expectant parents to navigate and manage severe morning sickness more effectively.

6. Ethical and Safety Considerations:

- Ethical Guidelines: Developing and adhering to stringent ethical guidelines ensuring the safety and well-being of pregnant individuals and their unborn children in any interventions or clinical trials related to morning sickness.

- Regulatory Frameworks: Formulating regulatory frameworks that balance the need for innovative treatments with stringent safety assessments in pregnancy-related therapies involving GDF15 modulation.

The future of managing severe morning sickness holds promise in targeted therapies, personalized medicine approaches, hormonal modulation, and lifestyle interventions. Ethical considerations, robust clinical trials, and comprehensive support systems will be critical in shaping these advancements and ensuring safe and effective treatments for pregnant individuals.

Chapter7:

Empowering Expectant Parents

Coping Mechanisms: Offering practical strategies and lifestyle adjustments to manage morning sickness symptoms

1. Dietary Modifications:

- Frequent, Small Meals: Eating smaller, more frequent meals throughout the day instead of large meals can help prevent an empty stomach, which often triggers nausea.
- Avoiding Trigger Foods: Identifying and avoiding foods or smells that trigger nausea can help alleviate symptoms.

2. Hydration and Fluid Intake:

- Sipping Fluids: Staying hydrated by sipping fluids like water, ginger tea, or clear broth throughout the day can ease nausea.
- Avoiding Large Amounts at Once: Drinking slowly and avoiding large volumes of liquids at once might help prevent nausea associated with excessive intake.

3. Rest and Stress Management:

- Adequate Rest: Ensuring adequate sleep and rest can help manage fatigue and potentially reduce nausea symptoms.
- Stress Reduction Techniques: Practicing relaxation techniques such as deep breathing, meditation, or yoga may help reduce stress-induced nausea.

4. Ginger and Herbal Remedies:

- Ginger Supplements or Tea: Some individuals find relief from nausea by consuming ginger supplements, ginger tea, or ginger-containing snacks.
- Herbal Remedies: Herbal remedies like peppermint or chamomile might provide relief for certain individuals; however, consulting a healthcare professional before use is advisable.

5. Acupressure and Alternative Therapies:

- Acupressure Bands: Using acupressure bands on the wrists or trying acupuncture might alleviate nausea symptoms for some pregnant individuals.
- Consulting a Specialist: Consulting a qualified alternative medicine practitioner for acupuncture or other therapies might provide relief.

6. Environmental Adjustments:

- Ventilation: Ensuring good ventilation and avoiding strong smells or odors can help reduce triggers for nausea.
- Fresh Air: Spending time outdoors or in well-ventilated spaces might alleviate symptoms for some individuals.

7. Medication and Professional Guidance:

- Consulting a Healthcare Professional: Seeking guidance from a healthcare provider regarding safe medications or supplements for managing severe morning sickness is crucial.
- Prescribed Medications: In severe cases, healthcare professionals might prescribe anti-nausea medications to alleviate symptoms. It's essential to follow their advice and guidelines.

8. Emotional Support and Understanding:

- Seeking Support Networks: Connecting with other expectant parents or support groups can

provide emotional support and shared experiences in coping with morning sickness.
- Communicating with Healthcare Providers: Keeping open communication with healthcare providers about the severity of symptoms and their impact on daily life is essential for tailored support and guidance.

While coping mechanisms and lifestyle adjustments can help manage morning sickness symptoms, it's crucial to individualize these strategies and consult healthcare professionals for personalized guidance, especially in cases of severe or persistent symptoms.

Supportive Measures: Providing emotional support and guidance for expectant parents navigating severe morning sickness

1. Open Communication:

- Encourage Open Dialogue: Foster an environment where the expectant parent feels comfortable discussing their experiences and the impact of severe morning sickness on their daily life.

- Active Listening: Provide a non-judgmental space for them to express their feelings, concerns, and challenges related to their condition.

2. <u>Emotional Support:</u>

- Offer Empathy and Understanding: Validate their experiences and emotions, acknowledging the difficulties they face due to severe morning sickness.
- Express Support: Show compassion, understanding, and reassurance that they are not alone in dealing with these challenging symptoms.

3. <u>Practical Assistance:</u>

- Assisting with Daily Tasks: Offer to assist with household chores, errands, or childcare responsibilities, recognizing that severe symptoms might limit their ability to carry out usual activities.
- Provide Rest Opportunities: Encourage and facilitate opportunities for adequate rest and relaxation whenever possible.

4. <u>Research and Information:</u>

- Educate and Inform: Provide access to reliable information about severe morning sickness, its potential causes, coping strategies, and available support networks.

- Understanding Treatment Options: Help in researching and understanding available treatment options or strategies for managing severe symptoms, while emphasizing the importance of consulting healthcare professionals.

5. Accompanying Medical Appointments:

- Support During Consultations: Accompany the expectant parent to medical appointments if possible, offering emotional support and assistance in addressing concerns or questions with healthcare providers.
- Ensuring Follow-ups: Assist in keeping track of appointments, follow-ups, and recommended treatments as advised by healthcare professionals.

6. Emotional Well-being:

- Encourage Self-care: Promote activities that foster emotional well-being, such as relaxation techniques, mindfulness exercises, or engaging in hobbies they enjoy.
- Seeking Professional Help: Encourage seeking professional help if severe morning sickness leads to emotional distress or mental health concerns.

7. Support Networks:

- Connecting with Others: Encourage participation in support groups or networks with other expectant parents facing similar challenges, fostering a sense of community and shared experiences.

8. Patience and Understanding:

- Be Patient: Understand that coping with severe morning sickness can be a prolonged process, and recovery may take time. Offer ongoing support and patience.

Supporting expectant parents dealing with severe morning sickness involves a compassionate and comprehensive approach that acknowledges the multifaceted challenges they face during this sensitive period of pregnancy.

Providing emotional support, understanding, and practical assistance can significantly impact the well-being of expectant parents navigating severe morning sickness. Creating a supportive environment and offering empathy can help alleviate the emotional burden of coping with challenging symptoms during pregnancy.

Chapter8:

Conclusion

Paving the Way Forward: Summarizing breakthroughs, challenges, and ongoing research in the realm of morning sickness treatment

<u>Breakthroughs:</u>

- GDF15 and Hormonal Pathways: Significant strides have been made in understanding the role of GDF15 and hormonal pathways, shedding light on their association with the onset and severity of morning sickness symptoms.
- Genetic Associations: Emerging research has identified genetic variations associated with heightened GDF15 levels pre-pregnancy, linking them to increased susceptibility to severe morning sickness, offering potential insights for targeted treatments.
- Clinical Trials and Interventions: Clinical trials exploring potential treatments targeting GDF15 modulation or hormonal pathways have shown promise in managing nausea and vomiting, although dedicated studies focusing specifically

on pregnancy-related morning sickness are still evolving.

<u>Challenges:</u>

- Complexity and Multifactorial Nature: Morning sickness is multifactorial, making it challenging to pinpoint specific causative factors or mechanisms. Understanding the interplay between genetics, hormones, and environmental factors remains intricate.
- Ethical and Safety Considerations: Altering GDF15 activity or exploring new treatments necessitates stringent ethical considerations, particularly regarding safety during pregnancy and potential effects on fetal development.
- Translation from Animal Studies to Human Treatments: While animal studies have shown promise, translating these findings to effective and safe treatments in humans, especially pregnant individuals, requires extensive research and clinical validation.

<u>Ongoing Research and Future Directions:</u>

- GDF15 Modulation and Targeted Therapies: Continued research aims to develop targeted therapies modulating GDF15 activity or related hormonal pathways specifically tailored for managing severe morning sickness during pregnancy.
- Genetic Profiling and Personalized Medicine: Advancements in genetic profiling aim to

identify individuals at higher risk for severe morning sickness, potentially paving the way for personalized interventions and treatments.

- Comprehensive Support Systems: Ongoing efforts focus on establishing comprehensive support systems involving healthcare professionals, support groups, and educational resources for expectant parents coping with severe morning sickness.

Breakthroughs in understanding GDF15, genetic associations, and hormonal pathways offer promising avenues for tailored treatments in managing severe morning sickness. However, challenges persist in translating research findings into safe and effective interventions, necessitating ongoing multidisciplinary research and comprehensive support frameworks.

Empowerment Through Knowledge: Encouraging informed decision-making and proactive approaches for expectant parents

1.<u>Comprehensive Understanding:</u>

- Education on Morning Sickness: Equipping expectant parents with comprehensive information about the nature, causes, and potential impacts of severe morning sickness enables informed decision-making.

2.<u>Access to Resources:</u>

- Reliable Information Sources: Providing access to trustworthy resources, such as reputable medical websites, books, or support groups, helps them gather accurate information and understand available options.

3.<u>Informed Decision-Making:</u>

- Discussing Treatment Options: Encouraging open discussions with healthcare providers about various treatment options, their benefits, risks, and potential outcomes empowers expectant parents to make informed choices.

4.<u>Advocating for Personal Needs:</u>

- Encouraging Active Participation: Encouraging expectant parents to actively engage in discussions with healthcare professionals, advocating for their needs, preferences, and concerns related to severe morning sickness.

5.Holistic Approaches:

- Exploring Multiple Strategies: Encouraging the exploration of multiple coping strategies, including lifestyle modifications, dietary changes, and potential treatments, while considering their effectiveness and safety.

6.Building a Support Network:

- Seeking Emotional Support: Encouraging expectant parents to seek emotional support from family, friends, or support groups, fostering a network of understanding and empathy during this challenging period.

7.Stress Management:

- Stress Reduction Techniques: Promoting stress management techniques like relaxation exercises, meditation, or engaging in activities they enjoy aids in coping with the emotional toll of severe morning sickness.

8.Preparing for Care and Recovery:

- Planning Ahead: Assisting in planning for care during periods of severe symptoms and preparing for gradual recovery, discussing lifestyle adjustments and resumption of regular activities post-recovery.

9.Importance of Follow-ups:

- Continued Communication: Emphasizing the importance of ongoing communication with healthcare providers, ensuring regular follow-ups, and monitoring progress during treatment.

10.Awareness of Options:

- Exploration of Alternative Therapies: Discussing alternative therapies or complementary approaches within safe and evidence-based frameworks, if desired, to complement conventional treatments.

The exploration of morning sickness, from its pervasive presence to the groundbreaking insights into its physiological underpinnings, has offered a multifaceted view of this complex phenomenon experienced by expectant parents worldwide. Beginning with an in-depth examination of the phenomenon itself, the outline delved into the physical, emotional, and social ramifications of morning sickness on expectant parents, shedding light on its far-reaching implications. The distinction between typical morning sickness and severe hyperemesis gravidarum provided a nuanced understanding, offering clarity in identifying and managing extreme cases.

Global prevalence rates highlighted the varying experiences across cultures, while the investigation into fetal hormones, especially GDF15, uncovered intriguing links to the onset and severity of morning sickness. Understanding GDF15's role, genetic associations, and potential therapeutic avenues offered hope for tailored treatments to mitigate its impact.

Insights from animal studies and clinical trials investigating GDF15's effects provided glimpses into potential future treatments, although ethical considerations and safety remain paramount in their development and application.

Addressing challenges and offering coping mechanisms and supportive measures underscored the importance of holistic care, emphasizing empathy, and practical assistance for expectant parents navigating severe morning sickness.

Encouraging informed decision-making and empowering expectant parents through knowledge and support emerged as a crucial theme, advocating for open dialogue, personalized care, and proactive approaches.

As research continues, the outline's conclusion reinforces the importance of a multidisciplinary approach, ongoing support systems, and the pursuit of safe, effective treatments to alleviate the burdens of severe morning sickness. It stands as a testament to the collaborative efforts needed to navigate this challenging yet hopeful terrain with compassion, understanding, and a relentless pursuit of solutions for the well-being of expectant parents and their precious bundles of joy.